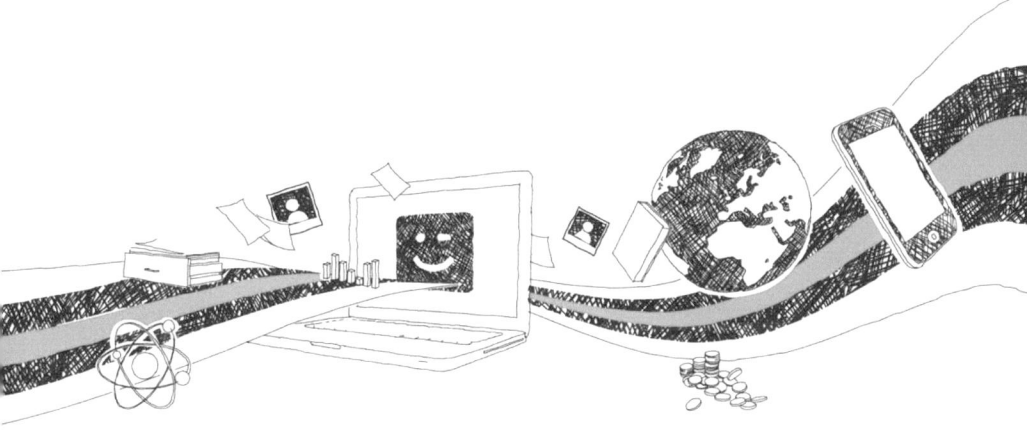
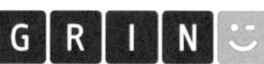

Bibliographic information published by the German National Library:

The German National Library lists this publication in the National Bibliography; detailed bibliographic data are available on the Internet at http://dnb.dnb.de .

Imprint:

Copyright © 2016 GRIN Verlag, Open Publishing GmbH
Print and binding: Books on Demand GmbH, Norderstedt Germany
ISBN: 978-3-668-13615-1

This book at GRIN:

http://www.grin.com/en/e-book/314444/modafinil-as-an-aid-to-reduce-tobacco-use-and-abuse

Joseph Parampathu

Modafinil as an aid to reduce tobacco use and abuse

GRIN Publishing

GRIN - Your knowledge has value

Since its foundation in 1998, GRIN has specialized in publishing academic texts by students, college teachers and other academics as e-book and printed book. The website www.grin.com is an ideal platform for presenting term papers, final papers, scientific essays, dissertations and specialist books.

Visit us on the internet:

http://www.grin.com/

http://www.facebook.com/grincom

http://www.twitter.com/grin_com

Contents

Abstract

Modafinil, first developed in France at Lafo Laboratories by Michael Jouvet, has become a respected treatement for narcolepsy and sleep disorders ranging from sleep apnea to shift work sleep disorder. It has been touted for its strength in promoting wakefulness through suppressing the desire to, or reducing the perception of need for, sleep. Though the precise mechanisms of action by which Modafinil elicits its effects remain unclear, we are most interested by its promise in acting to increase the presence of monoamine nuerotransmitters, such as dopamine, at synapses by binding to the reuptake site and blocking these neurotransmitter transporters while simultaneously inhibiting many of the transporters' subsequent actions, as this has been pointed to as a possible reasoning behind its ability to induce wakefulness as well as maintain low abuse potential (though it is worth mentioning that some users have reported slight euphoria on the first use, with varying results in achieving this feeling again). Though nicotine alone has been shown to have "relatively weak" addictive potential, it has been shown that properties of tobacco smoke act to inhibit monoamine oxidases (MAO) in such a way as to potentiate the addictive potential of nicotine dramatically. Further, nicotine, having effects on wakefulness, sleep, and appetite, all factors moderated by modafinil use, may have some overlapping or related physiology. We are seeking to explore the possibility that modafinil may be useful as a novel treatment for nicotine dependence in smokers who are attempting to quit or reduce their smoking levels.

Introduction

Modafinil is a relatively new drug prescribed most often to treat sleep disorders and manage wakefulness in otherwise healthy patients. The mechanisms of action and precise physiology behind its profound effects are not completely understood and require further study. We hope to provide evidence primarily through an analysis of its underlying physiological effects suggesting the possibility for its use as a means to help abstinent smokers or smokers who are trying to quit smoking with nicotine avoidance.

There has not been much published research on this specific topic, of modafinil's effects in nicotine dependence treatment, but there are available two small sample studies with conflicting results, each providing its case for increased research into this potential treatment method. Presented in order of publication, the first study, involving 19 smokers, regarded smokers being given modafinil orally and after 2 hours and 10 minutes, being administered a nicotine lozenge. The subjects were tested on various self-reported traits, notably reporting an increase in "drug strength" of the lozinge for those taking modafinil, but the study reports that modafinil had no effect on nicotine withdrawal symptoms. (30)

The second study was conducted on even fewer subjects, only 9, and comes to somewhat conflicting conclusions, relative to the previous study mentioned. The results of this study point to the combination of modafinil with nicotine replacement as a cessation aid having benefits for withdrawal symptoms. (31) It would be efficacious to study the effects of modafinil on tobacco cessation under controlled laboratory conditions as well as over a multiple-session period so as to more closely mimic modafinil's use in patients to which it is already being prescribed as well as the reality of the journey towards final elimination of tobacco use from the life of a smoker who has been persistently trying to quit.

Clinical Use of Modafinil

Modafinil is a wake-promoting agent most notably touted for its effects in ameliorating the symptoms of sleep deprivation or sleepiness in a way that is notably different than classical amphetamines in that it is not stimulating, but sleep-abating. (29) Modafinil has been quite confidently prescribed in cases for treating sleep disorders such as narcolepsy, sleep apnea, and work-shift disorder, as well as attention or learning disorders such as ADHD. Further, it has shown promise in treating depressive symptoms from bipolar disorder, in a trial excluding patients with stimulant-induced manias; a single dose may hasten recovery from general anesthesia after a surgical procedure; a single dose was helpful in allowing night workers the ability to attend a daytime lecture after work, but did not improve their ability to drive home and caused sleep disturbances, subsequently. (29) Modafinil has been researched for its effects in management of excessive sleepiness from Parkinson's disease, cognition in chronic fatigue, and cocaine addiction, with mixed results; these trials were all conducted in small sample sizes. There have been no documented cases of addiction or dependence, but it may have some abuse potential. (29)

Much of the data available points to its remarkable effects in subjects who are already sleep deprived and are using the drug with the hopes of staving off the tendency to fall asleep. Further, its effects on wakefulness and general sleep management have been shown to be quite powerful when used in conjunction with strategic, short naps to recuperate some energy during multiple day long dosages and wake-times. (28)

Psychomimetic Effects Of Modafinil

Modafinil users most commonly note feelings of increased wakefulness and feelings of normality as well as an improved sense of attention and other cognitive benefits. (16) It is most useful in treating episodes of excessive daytime sleepiness and its users have reported a sense of relief as well as improvements in general well-being.

The effects tend to settle in within 1-2 hours and often last 5-8 hours for frequent users, while infrequent users report effects up to 10-15 hours after administration (orally).

There have been conflicting reports of feelings of tolerance build up from users, but scientific evidence from research studies have tended to not support this claim. It would be wise to consider at least the idea that the drug has some loss of psychological dramaticism in its effect after long term use. (17) Professional poker player Paul Phillips reportedly used doses of 200-300mg for an extended period of time and believes that the effects attenuated overtime as his body became noticeably used to the chemical. (18) Most interestingly, from the anecdotal evidence, it would seem that there is little evidence for modafinil's potential to go beyond tolerance building and towards dependence or physical addiction. It would seem that users do not fall below their baseline ability when ceasing use after a long period of sustained use, as is the case with other psychostimulants like caffeine or amphetamines. (17) Regardless, modafinil's potential for abuse should still be viewed within the context of being at least psychologically addicting, as users often feel returning to their baseline level of productivity puts them at an unacceptable disadvantage to their chemically enhanced self.

Psychotomimetic Effects of Tobacco

The physical effects most commonly associated with tobacco use or nicotine exposure are stimulation and sedation, with the former being more common in low doses and the latter in high doses. This contradiction has been termed Nesbitt's Paradox, as Nesbitt noted that smokers' behave in a more relaxed way as their smoking-induced arousal increases. (19) Further, vasoconstriction and appetite suppression are common effects, with abnormal heartbeat and dizziness being exhibited in cases of high doses. (20)

The cognitive effects of nicotine use are thought acceleration; focus, memory, and motivation enhanvement; euphoria, sexual arousal, and compulsive redosing; and anxiety and anxiety suppression, the relationinship between the last pair of effects being similar to the Nesbitt Paradox, with anxiety being present as a response to the stimulatory effects of low dose nicotine, and anxiety suppression being present as a response to the sedatory effects of beta-endorphins released during high doses. (20)

Mechanism of Action

Orexins/Hypocretins

Orexins or hypocretins are neuropeptides that regulate arousal, wakefulness, and appetite. They are pivotal in understanding the underlying mechanisms of narcolepsy and other sleep disorders, similar to the ones which modafinil is prescribed to treat. Genetic knockout mice for orexins tend to exhibit signs of narcolepsy, or excessive uncontrollable daytime sleepiness. (1) Further, central dosage of orexins promotes wakefulness and the orexin system is thought to be largely functionally important in regulating energy expenditure as it relates to management of symptoms of sleepiness. Further evidence for orexins uses in sleep management is that monkeys deprived of sleep for periods of 30-36 hours and then injected with orexins show a lack of motivation to sleep as well as a reduction in overall tiredness. (2)

Because orexin-A receptors have been implicated as important to the motivation to drug seeking behavior, a study investigated its effects in moderating nicotine addictive behavior in rats given a selective antagonist for orexin-A. Nicotine self-administration as well as motivation to seek and obtain the drug decreased. The insula has been implicated in regulating feelings of craving, and contains orexin-A receptors; it has been reported that smokers who sustained damage to the insula lost the desire to smoke. (3)

Nicotine upregulates expression of orexin and its receptors at various locations in the brain. (5) Modafinil has been shown to actually be more effective in wakefulness promotion in rats that

5

have been genetically modified to have a nonfunctional orexin system than in baseline rats, which has been attributed to compensatory facilitation of central arousal through non-orexin based systems in these null mice, but the orexin system does seem to mediate some of the alerting effects of the drug. (6)

With respect to the orexin system it may be the case that the stimulation of orexin presence in the brain by modafinil is creating an environment similar to that elicited immediately after a user has administered their preferred dose of nicotine, during which the user is likely to exhibit feelings of being in a refractory period of being less sensitive to the desired effects of as well as less attracted by the notion of, administering the drug again. By saturating the brain with chemicals the user may only be used to feeling when already satisfied by their nicotine intake, the orexin system may be able to regulate the additional self-administration of nicotine to the point of reducing use for the duration of modafinil's effects. (4)

Histamine

The H1 receptor of histamine has been implicated in moderation of the sleep-wake cycle, nociception, regulation of appetite, and cognition. Further, the H3 receptor of histamine has modulates nociception as well as food intake among other things. (8) Modafinil has been shown to increase histamine production by 150% of the basal release. The i.c.v. injection of modafinil also yielded a similar increase in histamine production, but notably this production increase was not present from injection directly into the tuberomammillary nucleus, a region involved with arousal, learning, memory, and sleep, where histaminergic neurons are largely present. (9)

Nicotine seems to have in one role an antagonistic relation with histamine when the nicotine is present in high doses. Further, it would seem that in low doses, nicotine has a residually inhibitory effect on histamines. This second effect has been attributed to a refractoriness incident of a combination of nicotine-induced paralysis of ganglion cells which mediate histamine release and an after-effect of the contraction of the gut or the release of acetylcholine which lead to the contraction. (7)

It has been shown that nicotine agonists inhibit the release of histamines from human basophilis white blood cells. (10) It may be the case that in response to the neuronal environment of increased histaminergic activity and the general feelings of wakefulness such an environment promotes, the body's cravings for a histamine release-reducing chemical to which it is already

6

accustomed to, such as nicotine through tobacco in the bodies of smokers, is reduced and the smoker's appetite for nicotine administration is mediated through this pharmaco-cognitive relationship.

Dopamine

The mesocorticolimbic dopaminergic (DA) system is a series of projections beginning in the ventral tegmental area (VTA) and innervating the striatum, amygdala, and prefrontal cortex that is highly implicated in the motivation of addictive behavior and learning as it relates to drugs of abuse such as nicotine, cocaine, and amphetamines. Increases of available DA in the systems of the mesocorticolimbic system like the nucleus accumbens have been long associated with the positive reinforcement of administration of these drugs that leads to their high abuse potential and possible addiction. (11)

There is evidence that the DA acts to convey novelty and errors in reward signaling, as the firing of DA neurons reflects the difference between expected and actual reward. It would seem that this moderation of previous experience to present stimuli creates the environment for complex learning. (13) The mesocorticolimbic system as a whole acts to integrate knowledge of previous interactions with salient environmental information. (12) The DA system provides the context with which an animal or human can act to respond to potentially rewarding stimuli such as food or sex to enforce long term survivability. (14)

Dopaminergic neurotransmission is reduced during nicotine withdrawal. Nicotine addiction abatement programs that focus on DA neurotransmission act to alleviate the symptoms of withdrawal. (15) With regards to the effects of modafinil as a dopaminergic agent, there may be promise for modafinil as a method for increasing the DA levels to that above what we expect in humans or animals experiencing withdrawal symptoms which put them in a state vulnerable to nicotine self-administration or similar drug seeking behavior. Thus the user may be relieved of the compulsion or desire to smoke when under the influence of modafinil.

Glutamate

Glutamate has been Implicated as playing a subtle role in the alertness effects of modafinil and seems to generally raise extracellular glutamate levels. Modafinil is thought to elicit this effect by blocking receptor activity such that glutamate is not absorbed by the postsynaptic neuron, allowing glutamate levels at the synapse to build dramatically. (22)

During prolonged abstinence the hypoglutaminergic neuronal state plays a role in enforcing nicotine-seeking behavior. (21) Modafinil may play a role in raising this hypoglutaminergic state back to baseline so as to mitigate the effects of nicotine withdrawal which provide the environment that enforces nicotine-seeking behavior.

Glutamate release in the VTA excites release of DA, producing the rewarding effects of nicotine use. It is suggested that smoking cessation can be facilitated by the reduction of glutamate transmission which decreases the reward elicited by nicotine use. (23) Modafinil may show promise in this regard by blocking the uptake of glutamate at the postsynaptic neuron, thus blocking the rewarding DA release expected from nicotine use. This difference between expected and actual reward is pivotal in addiction learning and relearning as well as extinction reponses. By "reprogramming" the brain to no longer associate the nicotine use with nicotine, through DA, reward, modafinil may be providing an effective, possibly long-term improvement to a user's relationship to nicotine as a drug of dependence.

Immediate withdrawal symptoms are a key mechanism in the dependence and abuse potential of tobacco products, particularly when smoked. After nicotine exposure, as the effects of nicotine withdrawal set in, synaptic glutamate depletion occurs. This glutamate depletion is and related withdrawal symptoms are implicated as a major cause behind the motivation to immediate redosing with nicotine. (24) Medications that increase synaptic glutamate levels may help to alleviate the symptoms of nicotine withdrawal and reduce to craving to smoke in abstinent smokers. (25)

Glutamate transmission plays a role in extinction learning, the process of erasing or rewriting old reward associations with new ones. (26) By creating an environment rich with glutamate, modafinil use may be bringing the brain to a stage that is effective for relearning associations that have been ingrained over long periods of time, such as smoking dependence reactions. Administration of compounds to increase or facilitate glutaminergic compounds have been presented as a strategy to prevent relapse in abstinent smokers by encouraging extinction and relearning. (25)

Animals show depressive-like symptoms during withdrawal from chronic nicotine exposure during abstinence that has been linked to decreased glutaminergic transmission. NMDA receptor antagonists, which lower glutaminergic transmission, can reduce the reinforcing effects of nicotine. (27) It should be noted, modafinil is considered to be a partial NMDA agonist, so its moderating effects on the glutaminergic system through NMDA receptor binding may be conflicted.

Conclusions and Suggestions for Future Research

It would seem that there are multiple and sometimes conflicting mechanisms by which modafinil may be effective in promoting nicotine avoidance during smoking cessation. Truly, the methods by which modafinil affects a patient's physiology are complex and wide-reaching in their physiological effects, even while being meticulously specific in other regards. The most promising pathways by which these effects seem to present themselves are through the expression of orexins, or hypocretins, glutamate, and histamines, while having further less pronounced or less specific effects regarding dopamine, serotonin, GABA, and MAO. Further study on these specific relationships within a context of coming to understand the potential for modafinil to act as a moderating agent in nicotine self-administration during smoking abstinence may prove to be useful.

We would suggest the most operationally useful studies would take place over longer periods of time within smokers who are trying to quit but have been unsuccessful and are open to the use of aids in smoking cessation therapy to be used either in conjunction with total abstinence or nicotine replacement therapy, under double-blind conditions, testing against a control for placebo effect. We suggest that these smokers be monitored or self-report their smoking habits during this time that they are attempting to avoid smoking, so that we can compare this data to their previous success in quitting or reducing their smoking habits.

Sources

1. https://www.ncbi.nlm.nih.gov/pubmed/10481909

2. https://www.ncbi.nlm.nih.gov/pubmed/18160631

3. http://www.sciencedaily.com/releases/2008/11/081124174851.htm

4. https://www.wpi.edu/Pubs/E-project/Available/E-project-042408-112010/unrestricted/MQP_REPORT_Zand_Angjeli.pdf

5. http://www.ncbi.nlm.nih.gov/pubmed/11014216

6. http://www.ncbi.nlm.nih.gov/pubmed/15652995

7. http://onlinelibrary.wiley.com/store/10.1111/j.1476-5381.1951.tb00620.x/asset/j.1476-5381.1951.tb00620.x.pdf;jsessionid=E0E59E093D0BCB2CBFE35C9FA93F2607.f01t04?v=1&t=ijknzl3s&s=49bb310f17523fe19d504dcc17754d27d127f007

8. https://www.ncbi.nlm.nih.gov/pubmed/26084539

9. http://www.ncbi.nlm.nih.gov/pubmed/12614915/

10. http://link.springer.com/article/10.1007%2Fs00011-004-1249-1

11. http://www.ncbi.nlm.nih.gov/pubmed/3317472

12. http://www.ncbi.nlm.nih.gov/pubmed/10078530

13. http://www.ncbi.nlm.nih.gov/pubmed/8774460

14. http://www.jneurosci.org/content/22/9/3306.long

15. http://www.ncbi.nlm.nih.gov/pmc/articles/PMC3188825/

16. http://ajp.psychiatryonline.org/doi/full/10.1176/ajp.158.8.1341

17. http://www.gwern.net/Modafinil

18. http://www.newyorker.com/magazine/2009/04/27/brain-gain

19. http://www.ncbi.nlm.nih.gov/pubmed/6741672

20. http://www.ncbi.nlm.nih.gov/pubmed/2560221

21. http://www.ncbi.nlm.nih.gov/pubmed/16876138/

22. http://www.nature.com/npp/journal/v20/n4/full/1395268a.html

23. http://www.ncbi.nlm.nih.gov/pubmed/10900219/

24. http://www.ncbi.nlm.nih.gov/pubmed/19103434/

25. http://www.ncbi.nlm.nih.gov/pmc/articles/PMC3188825/

26. http://www.ncbi.nlm.nih.gov/pubmed/20631689/

27. http://www.ncbi.nlm.nih.gov/pubmed/18418357/

28. http://www.dtic.mil/dtic/tr/fulltext/u2/p011050.pdf
29. http://www.ncbi.nlm.nih.gov/pubmed/18729534
30. http://www.ncbi.nlm.nih.gov/pubmed/17868195
31. http://www.ncbi.nlm.nih.gov/pmc/articles/PMC4120247/

YOUR KNOWLEDGE HAS VALUE

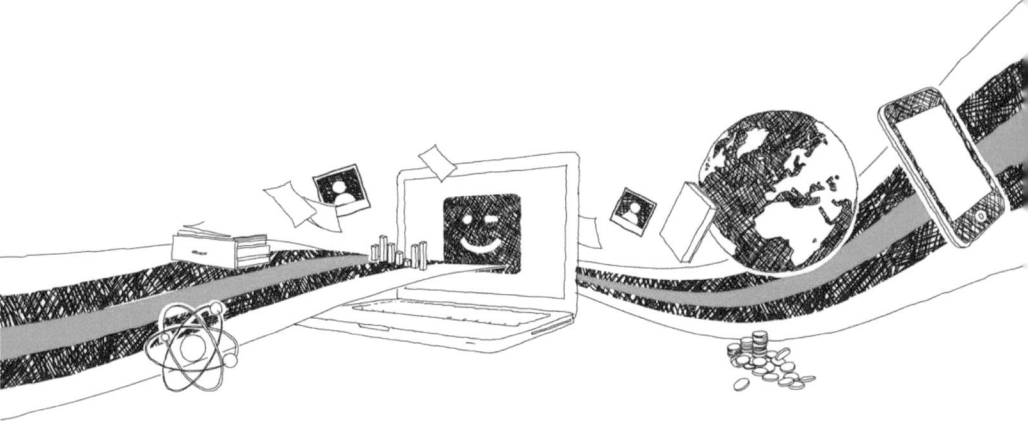

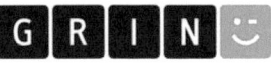